PRINCIPLES OF INFECTION CONTROL PRACTICE

Edited by

Anne Griffiths-Jones
BSc (Hons) RGN DipN (Lond) Infection
Control Nurse, Glan Hafren NHS Trust

and

Kate Ward
RN, RSCN, FETC Specialist Nurse
Adviser, Public Health, Southern
Derbyshire Health Authority

Scutari Press

© Scutari Press 1995

Scutari Press is a division of Scutari Projects Ltd,
the publishing company of the Royal College of Nursing.

First published 1995

British Library Cataloguing in Publication Data

Principles of Infection Control Practice,
  I. Griffiths-Jones, Anne   II. Ward, Kate
  614.44

  ISBN 1-873853-05-x

Typesetting by Dorwyn Ltd, Rowlands Castle, Hants
Printed and bound in Great Britain by Hobbs the Printers of Southampton

PRINCIPLES
OF
INFECTION
CONTROL
PRACTICE

Editors

Anne Griffiths-Jones
Kate Ward

CONTRIBUTORS

Gill Beaumont
FIBMS

Infection Control Liaison Officer, Kingsmill Centre for Health Care Services, Mansfield, Nottingham

Andrea Buckles
RGN, DipN (Lond)

Infection Control Nurse, Royal Liverpool University Hospital

Andrew Crawford
RMN, RGN, ADN
(Infection Control)

Infection Control Nursing Officer, Renfrew Priority Services, Paisley

Anne Crawford
RGN, SCM, ADN
(Infection Control)

Clinical Nurse Specialist, Infection Control, Vale of Leven District General Hospital

Eilish Creamer
RGN, RM

Infection Control Sister, Beaumont Hospital, Dublin

Dee Dearden
RGN, DMS

Senior Nurse Infection Control, Queens Medical Centre, Nottingham

Beryl Donaldson
RGN, SCM, FETC

Senior Nurse Infection Control, Royal Victoria Infirmary, Newcastle-Upon-Tyne

Anne Griffiths-Jones
BSc (Hons), RGN,
DipN (Lond)

Infection Control Nurse, Glan Hafren NHS Trust

Paul Hateley
RGN, RMN, OND

Senior Nurse Infection Control, St Bartholomew's Hospital, London

Dawn Hill
RGN, ONC

Clinical Nurse Specialist, Infection Control, Dudley Road Hospital, Birmingham

PRINCIPLES
OF
INFECTION
CONTROL
PRACTICE

CONTENTS

INTRODUCTION

The primary aim of an infection control programme, whether in the community or hospital, is to prevent people from acquiring avoidable infection. Achieving this aim requires the willingness of all health care staff to maintain the highest possible standards of clinical practice and follow sound infection control principles. Unfortunately there are, even today, some methods used to control infection which are based on tradition but which have little effect on cross-infection rates.

Many health care workers have been involved, particularly over the last few years, in the setting of standards for clinical practice. Where the standards required infection control input, the Infection Control Nurse was often asked to contribute. However, situations have occurred where this advice has neither been sought nor been available. The Infection Control Nurses Association (ICNA) was asked to address this problem. After discussion it was agreed that the publication of a series of principles to provide a well-researched basis for infection control practice would be of most benefit to health care workers in a wide variety of specialties. It was recognised by the ICNA that, while there may be some diversity in practice, the principles on which actions are based should always display a degree of uniformity.

These broad principles of practice were written by Infection Control Nurses in England, Wales, Scotland and Ireland. Each set was sent to all the other groups for peer review and therefore represent a consensus of opinion. It is hoped that the contents of this book will provide not only a valuable source of information which will aid in the setting and maintenance of nursing standards but will also provide a starting point to bring about change. It should be noted that the first principle, Rights of Individuals, should form the foundation on which all the remaining principles are built.

1 RIGHTS OF INDIVIDUALS

Definition The term describes Infection Control procedures which are designed to embrace the physical, social, spiritual and psychological needs of individuals and their families.

Aim To introduce a holistic approach to Infection Control practices which becomes an integral part of nursing care.

Broad Principles

1. All individuals have the right to be protected from preventable infections (DHSS/PHLS 1988).

2. All individuals, whenever possible, have the right to be fully involved with, and understand the need for Infection Control procedure and policies (Grazier 1988).

3. An individual's privacy and dignity should be maintained throughout any Infection Control procedure.

4. All individuals should have access to members of the Infection Control Team.

5. All individuals have the right to expect Infection Control procedures to be research-based (Thomlinson 1990).

6. All individuals should have an opportunity to participate in an Infection Control education programme (Caddow 1989).

7. All individuals should have the right to expect adequate resources to be made available for comprehensive Infection Control programmes.

References

Caddow P (ed) (1989) *Applied Microbiology.* London: Scutari Press.

DHSS/PHLS Hospital Infection Working Group (1988) *Hospital Infection Control: Guidance on the Control of Infection in Hospitals.* London: HMSO.

Grazier S (1988) The loneliness barrier. *Nursing Times* **84**(41): 44–45.

Thomlinson D (1990) Time to dispense with the rituals. *Professional Nurse* **5**(8): 421–425.

2 HANDWASHING

Definition Describes a process which removes potentially pathogenic organisms from the hands.

Aim Prevent hands becoming a vehicle of cross-
infection.

Broad Principles

1. The friction caused by rubbing and rinsing the hands, coupled with
the rough action of paper towels, should physically remove microorganisms (Gould 1992).

2. Handwashing or disinfecting technique, regardless of the product
selected must ensure no area of skin surface is missed during the
procedure (Ayliffe et al. 1992).

3. Resources used for handwashing must not create a cross-infection
hazard, e.g.

   3.1 Poorly cleaned and maintained hand basins and soap dispen-
   sers (Bowell 1992).

   3.2 Bar soap left in containers where moisture can accumulate
   (Bowell 1992).

   3.3 Communal hand towels (Sneddon 1990).

4. Patients should have access to handwashing facilities particularly
following the use of a bed pan or commode (Bowell 1992).

5. Nail brushes can damage the skin and increase the risk of colonisa-
tion with potentially pathogenic organisms. Their continued use is
therefore inadvisable (Ayliffe et al. 1992).

6. The frequency of handwashing and method selected should reflect
risks of cross-infection and facilities available.

   6.1 *Low Risk (social handwash with soap and water)*
   • Undertaken prior to most ward procedures.

6.2 *Medium/High Risk (hygienic hand disinfection using an anti-microbial preparation)*
- Undertaken in special units, e.g. ITU, SCBU, isolation units, prior to any aseptic procedure.
- Indicated during outbreaks of infection.

6.3 *High Risk (surgical hand disinfection using an antimicrobial preparation: Longer contact time (2 minutes) than 6.2*
- Prior to wearing sterile clothing.
- Prior to any surgical intervention (Ayliffe et al. 1992).

6.4 The wearing of gloves is not a substitute for handwashing.

6.5 Damage to the skin may be caused by failure to rinse hands properly or by inadequate drying technique (Meers et al. 1992).

References

Ayliffe GAJ, Lowbury EJL, Geddes AM and Williams JD (1992) *Control of Hospital Infection – A Practical Handbook*, 3rd Edition. London: Chapman & Hall.

Bowell B (1992) Hands up for cleanliness. *Nursing Standard* 6(15/16): 24–25.

Gould D (1992) Hygienic hand decontamination. *Nursing Standard* 6(32): 33–36.

Meers P, Jacobsen W and McPherson M (1992) *Hospital Infection Control for Nurses*. London: Chapman & Hall.

Sneddon JG (1990) A preventable course of infection. *Professional Nurse* 6(2): 92–104.

3 ISOLATION NURSING

(a) SOURCE ISOLATION

Definition Precautions taken to prevent the spread of an organism to any individual from a patient with a transmissible infection.

Aim To confine the organism or block its route of spread (Taylor 1981).

(b) PROTECTIVE ISOLATION

Definition Precautions taken to protect susceptible patients from exogenous infections.

Aim To prevent the transfer of infective microorganisms to patients at special risk from infection.

Broad Principles

1. By attending to psychological needs, the patient's feelings of stress and anxiety should be minimised during the isolation procedure (Denton 1986).

2. When planning patient care, individualised patient needs should be balanced against recognised modes of transmission, e.g. if an infection is spread by the airborne route, the door of a cubicle or side room should be kept closed (Gould 1987).

3. Meticulous hand hygiene (*see* Principle No. 2) should be taken to prevent hands from becoming a vehicle for cross-infection (Ayliffe et al. 1992).

4. When a single room is necessary, it should have sufficient resources to facilitate infection control practices, e.g. toilet, handwash basin (Meers et al. 1992).

5. The equipment used, where practical, should be either disposable or autoclavable (Ayliffe et al. 1992).

6. Contaminated crockery and cutlery should be adequately disinfected, e.g. in a hot dishwasher cycle with a minimum temperature of 60°C and a final rinse of 82°C (Griffiths 1990).

7. All clinical waste should be disposed of safely (*see* Principle No. 12).

8. Linen contaminated with potentially hazardous blood or body fluids should be transported safely to the laundry in accordance with local agreed policy, e.g. inner water soluble bag; outer red plastic bag which should be securely tied (Department of Health 1987).

9. In both categories of isolation nursing, protective clothing should be worn to prevent cross-infection from recognised routes of transmission (Wilson 1992), e.g.
   9.1 Impermeable plastic apron to protect the uniform (Gill and Slater 1991).
   9.2 Disposable non-sterile latex gloves, if contact with infectious material or potentially infected material is anticipated.
   9.3 Eye-wear, when there is a risk of splashing into eyes from blood or body fluids.
   9.4 Masks are of limited value but may be recommended in specific situations to prevent the spread of respiratory-borne infection. If worn, masks should be of the filter type and fit closely to the contours of the face.

10. Protective clothing should not become a source of cross infection, therefore clothes should be discarded and hands washed immediately after attending to all the patient's needs (Wilson 1992).

11. An assessment should be made on whether relatives wear protective clothing based on the risk of infection to themselves and the patients.

12. The environment should not become a source of cross-infection, therefore the importance of regular domestic cleaning and immediate removal of spillage of body fluids remains paramount (Wilson 1992).

References

Ayliffe GAJ, Lowbury EJL, Geddes AM and Williams JD (1992) *Control of Hospital Infection: A Practical Handbook*, 3rd Edition. London: Chapman & Hall.

Department of Health (1987) *Hospital Laundry Arrangements for Used and Infected Linen.* HC(87)30. London: HMSO.

Denton PF (1986) Psychological and physiological effect of isolation. *Nursing* **3**(3): 88–91.

Gill J and Slater J (1991) Building barriers against infection. *Nursing Times* **87**(50): 53–54.

Gould D (1987) *Infection and Patient Care.* London: Heinemann.

Griffiths G (1990) Principles of Isolation Nursing. In: Worsley MA, Ward KA and Parker L (eds) *Infection Control Guidelines for Nursing Care.* Livingston: ICNA/Surgikos.

Meers P, Jacobsen W and McPherson M (1992) *Hospital Infection Control for Nurses.* London: Chapman & Hall.

Taylor LJ (1981) Isolation and barrier nursing. *Nursing* **1**(29): 1267–1269.

Wilson J (1992) Theory and practice of isolation nursing. *Nursing Standard* **6**(17): 30–31.

4 INTRAVENOUS CARE

Definition A collective term which is used to describe the management of patients undergoing some form of intravascular cannulation.

Aims (i) To prevent both exogenous and endogenous infections.
(ii) To observe for post-cannulation complications.

Broad Principles

1. The principles of asepsis (see Principle No. 5) should be adhered to during the insertion, management and removal of the cannula, administration of **any** intravenous therapy and inspection of the insertion site (Gould 1987).

2. Effective handwashing remains the most important means of preventing infection. This should be undertaken prior to the insertion of any intravenous (IV) cannula, handling of the cannula as well as preceding any further handling of the administration set (Maki 1991).

3. Protective clothing should be worn in relation to any local Blood and Body Fluid Precautions guidelines. Consideration should be given to staff wearing **sterile** gloves when inserting the cannula for any immunocompromised patient (Goodinson 1990).

4. The selected site should be **visibly** clean before a broad-spectrum skin disinfectant, such as 70% alcohol with or without chlorhexidine or povidone-iodine, is applied and allowed to dry (Ayliffe et al. 1992).

5. The infusion bag/bottle should be checked for expiry date and the existence of faults, such as leaks or cloudiness, before connecting to the giving set. If any are present or if the fluid is out of date, it must be discarded or returned to pharmacy in accordance with local agreed policy (Ayliffe et al. 1992).

6. After insertion, the intravenous device should be firmly secured to prevent any movement which could aid the entry of microorganisms (Goodinson 1990). Immediately after use, sharps should safely be disposed of in an appropriate container.

7. The infusion site should be kept clean and dry and assessed for any evidence of complications such as infection or phlebitis (Alderman 1988).

8. A sterile dressing should cover the insertion site. This could be either a sterile gauze or a transparent polyurethane dressing. This dressing should be changed weekly, when damaged or if fluid collects around the insertion site (Wilson 1994).

9. The frequency of changing administration sets should not exceed that which is supported by current knowledge (Collins and Josse 1987), e.g.:
   - Giving sets: changed every 48–72 hours or immediately after giving blood or lipids.
   - Infusion bags or bottles: changed every 12–24 hours.
   - Peripheral cannulae: changed every 48–72 hours (if another appropriate site is available).
   - Peripheral cannulae should be immediately removed if there is any sign or symptoms of infection. The tip should be sent to the laboratory for culture (Ayliffe et al. 1992).

10. A closed system should be maintained. Therefore three-way taps, stopcocks or similar devices should be avoided whenever possible (Speechley 1984).

11. If phlebitis or infection is suspected, the Medical or Intravenous Therapy Team should be informed.

References

Alderman C (1988) Practical aspects of intravenous infusion. *Nursing Standard* 2(49):
26–27.

Ayliffe GAJ, Lowbury EJL, Geddes AM and
Williams JD (1992) *Control of Hospital Infec-
tion – A Practical Handbook*, 3rd Edition.
London: Chapman & Hall.

Collins BJ and Josse ED (1987) Infection in
intensive therapy units. *Care of the Critically
Ill* 3(1): 3–5.

Goodinson S (1990) Keeping the flora out.
Professional Nurse 5(11): 572–575.

Gould D (1987) *Infection and Patient Care – A
Guide for Nurses*. London: Heinemann
Nursing.

Maki DG (1991) *Improving Catheter Site Care.
Proceedings of a Symposium sponsored by Smith
& Nephew Medical*. London: Royal Society
of Medicine.

Speechley V (1984) The nurse's role in intravenous management. *Nursing Times* 80(18):
31–32.

Wilson J (1994) Preventing infection during IV
therapy. *Professional Nurse* 9(6): 388–392.

5 ASEPSIS

Definition A collective term for the methods used to prevent microbial contamination of living tissue, fluids or sterile materials.

Aim (a) To prevent contamination of wounds and other susceptible sites.
(b) To prevent exogenous infection.

Broad Principles

1. The handwashing principle should be adhered to (*see* Principle No. 2). Following the first handwash, alcohol hand-rub should be available for use at any time during the procedure, particularly when unsterile articles have been touched (Ayliffe et al. 1992).

2. The patient's full involvement and cooperation must be sought, whenever practically possible, prior to any aseptic procedure (Boore 1979).

3. Nurse uniforms should not become a source of cross-infection, therefore they should be changed if wet or soiled.

4. The period of time during which microbial contamination of the site or equipment/materials may occur must be kept to a minimum (Ayliffe et al. 1992).

5. Any visible contamination must be removed according to local spillage/disinfection policy prior to the use of the trolley/surface area which is to be used for the aseptic technique.

6. All instruments, fluids and materials must be sterile. Packs should be checked to ensure that there is no evidence of damage or moisture penetration (Lascelles 1982).

7. A disposable plastic apron should be worn for each patient prior to commencing an aseptic procedure (Caddow 1990).

8. A significantly better wound or skin cleanse may be obtained when sterile gloved hands rather than forceps are used for an aseptic technique (Thomlinson 1987).

9. Where possible staff should be free of infection, e.g. colds, sore throats, septic lesions. Their fitness for duty may need to be assessed by the Occupational Health Staff or General Practitioner. Staff should ensure that any cuts or abrasions on their hands or forearms are covered with an occlusive dressing (Ayliffe et al. 1992).

10. Used equipment and waste should be dealt with according to local agreed policy (Collins and Josse 1990).

References

Ayliffe GAJ, Lowbury EJL, Geddes AM and Williams JD (1992) *Control of Hospital Infection. A Practical Handbook*, 3rd Edition. London: Chapman & Hall.

Boore JPR (1979) *Prescription for Recovery: The Effect of Pre-operative Preparation of Surgical Patients on Post-operative Stress, Recovery and Infection.* London: Royal College of Nursing.

Caddow P (ed) (1990) *Applied Microbiology.* London: Scutari Press.

Collins BJ and Josse ED (1990) The Patient's Environment. In: Worsley MA, Ward KA and Parker L (eds) *Infection Control Guidelines for Nursing Care.* Livingston: ICNA/Surgikos.

Lascelles I (1982) Wound dressing techniques. *Nursing* 8(2): 217–219.

Thomlinson D (1987) To clean or not to clean? *Nursing Times* 83(9), *The Journal of Infection Control Nursing*, 71–75.

6 WOUND CARE

Definition The application of the principles of asepsis when covering a patient's wound.

Aims (a) To promote healing.
(b) To minimise the risk of exogenous infection.

Broad Principles

1. Apply principles of asepsis (*see* Principle No. 5).

2. The wound dressing should be removed carefully to prevent dispersal of organisms (Ayliffe et al. 1992).

3. If the wound is clean and dry it is better to leave it alone and not attempt to clean it further (Thomlinson 1987).

4. If 'strike-through' occurs (i.e. leakage reaches the surface of the dressing) the dressing should be removed and a new one applied. Extra padding should not be applied over the soaked dressing (Ayliffe et al. 1992).

5. Avoid unnecessary prolonged exposure of wounds during dressing changes (David 1986).

6. Irrigation is the preferred method of cleansing wounds (Westaby 1985). Some materials, e.g. cotton wool and non-woven gauze may shed fibres into the wound and act as a focus for infection (Wood 1976).

7. Wounds should be cleaned using normal saline. The use of antiseptics can be injurious to tissues, hence caution in their use is advisable (Deas et al. 1986).

8. An accurate recording of the condition of the wound and skin should be made at each dressing change (Morrison 1987). This will aid the early detection of wound infection.

References

Ayliffe GAJ, Geddes AM, Lowbury EJL and Williams JD (1992) *Control of Hospital Infection – A Practical Handbook*, 3rd Edition. London: Chapman & Hall.

David JA (1986) *Wound Management. A Comprehensive Guide to Dressing and Healing.* London: Martin Dunnitz Ltd.

Deas J, Billings P and Brennan S (1986) The toxicity of commonly used antiseptics on fibroblasts in tissue culture. *Phlebology* 1(1): 205–209.

Morrison MJ (1987) Wound assessment. *Professional Nurse* 2(10): 315–317.

Thomlinson D (1987) To clean or not to clean? *Nursing Times* 83(9), *The Journal of Infection Control Nursing*, 71–75.

Westaby S (1985) *Wound Care.* London: Heinemann.

Wood RAB (1976) Disintegration of cellulose dressings in open granulating wounds. *British Medical Journal* 1(6023): 1444–5.

7 SPECIMEN COLLECTION

Definition The principles cover the collection of **any** specimens for laboratory investigation.

Aims (a) Collection of the requested specimen in an appropriate container with minimal risk of contamination.

(b) The immediate transfer of specimen to the laboratory.

Broad Principles

(a) REQUESTING A SPECIMEN

The request form must be completed accurately with the appropriate and relevant clinical details (Ayton 1982).

(b) COLLECTION OF SAMPLE

1. Local policies on protective clothing must be adhered to. Gloves, if worn, must be latex and conform to TSS/D/300.010 (ACP 1990).

2. The procedure of obtaining the specimen must not expose the patient to an increased risk of infection (Caddow 1989).

3. Specimens are required which are most appropriate for the clinical condition (Shanson 1989).

4. The specimen should not be contaminated by the normal flora of the patient or the member of staff (Caddow 1989).

5. It must be ensured that the specimen container is appropriate, that the specimen is safely contained and clearly labelled and that the container is not externally contaminated (HSAC 1991). The isolation of the organism is dependent on the quality of the specimen (Ayton 1982).

6. Any specimen known or suspected of presenting an infection hazard must be correctly labelled by the person requesting the laboratory investigation to allow identification (HSAC 1991).

7. The container should not be overfilled (filling the container to three quarters full is usually adequate) (Ayton 1982).

8. Prompt delivery to the laboratory should be ensured. If long delays are expected, specimens may need to be placed in transport medium (McFarlane 1989).

9. All specimens must be transported to the laboratory in an individual transparent plastic bag (HSAC 1991).

10. If a specimen container is found to be leaking or broken, a senior member of staff should be asked to deal with it in accordance with local agreed policy (HSAC 1991).

References

Advisory Committee on Dangerous Pathogens (1990) *The Causative Agent of AIDS and Related Conditions.* London: HMSO.

Ayton M (1982) Microbiological investigations. *Nursing* 2(8): 226–230.

Caddow P (ed) (1989) *Applied Microbiology.* London: Scutari Press.

Health Service Advisory Committee (1991) *Safety in Health Service Laboratories.* London: HMSO.

McFarlane A (1989) Using the laboratory in infection control. *Professional Nurse* 4(8): 393–397.

Shanson D (1989) *Microbiology in Clinical Practice*, 2nd Edition. Bristol: Wright.

8 PREOPERATIVE CARE

Definition Preoperative care is the physical and psychological preparation of the patient prior to surgery.

Aim To minimise the risk of the patient acquiring both endogenous and exogenous infection.

Broad Principles

1. The environment should be clean, well ventilated and well maintained (Ayliffe et al. 1991).

2. All equipment should not only be well maintained but also cleaned and disinfected or sterilised in accordance to local agreed policy (Ayliffe et al. 1992).

3. Factors which predispose to patients acquiring an infection should be minimised; consider the following examples:
   (a) Short preoperative hospital stay (Cruse and Foord 1980).
   (b) Assess the patient for history of infection or predisposing factors (Johnson 1989).
   (c) Optimise nutritional state (Holmes 1986).

4. Skin preparation should be carried out to reduce skin flora (Lowbury et al. 1988). The value of a preoperative bath has not been proven, although the dirt removing process is an important step prior to disinfection (MacKenzie 1988). Removal of hair should only be necessary to prevent interference with surgery. This procedure should be undertaken immediately prior to surgery (MacKenzie 1988).

5. Shaving can contribute to infection from organisms both endogenous and exogenous in origin. By disturbing skin scales and abrading skin it can increase the wound infection rate (Cruse and Foord

1973). Here, the use of depilatory creams (Seropian and Reynolds 1971) or clipping (Alexander et al. 1983) is advocated.

6. Patients requiring bowel surgery should have as much faecal matter as possible removed before surgery (Shanson 1983).

7. Antibiotic prophylaxis, which is the responsibility of medical staff, can reduce the wound sepsis rates if the appropriate agents are administered selectively (Shanson 1983).

8. Used equipment and waste should be dealt with in accordance with local agreed policies (Collins and Josse 1990).

9. All invasive procedures prior to surgery should be carried out applying the principles of asepsis (*see* Principle No. 5).

References

Ayliffe GAJ, Collins BJ and Taylor LJ (1991) *Hospital Acquired Infection. Principles and Prevention*, 2nd Edition. Guildford: Butterworth Heinemann Ltd.

Ayliffe GAJ, Lowbury EJL, Geddes AM and Williams JD (1988) *Control of Hospital Infection – A Practical Handbook*, 2nd Edition. London: Chapman & Hall.

Alexander JW, Fischer JE, Boyajain M, Palaiquist J and Morris MJ (1983) The influence of hair removal methods on wound infection. *Archives of Surgery* 118(3): 347–352.

Collins BJ and Josse ED (1990) The Patient's Environment. In: Worsley MA, Ward KA and Parker L (eds) *Infection Control Guidelines for Nursing Care*. Livingston: ICNA/Surgikos.

Cruse PJE and Foord A (1980) The epidemiology of wound infection – a ten year prospective study of 62 939 wounds. *Surgical Clinics of North America* 60(1): 27–40.

Cruse PJE and Foord A (1973) A five year prospective study of 23 649 surgical wounds. *Archives of Surgery* 107(2): 206–10.

Holmes S (1986) Nutritional needs of surgical patients. *Nursing Times* 5(44): 30–32.

Johnson A (1989) Preparing for elective surgery. *Nursing Standard* 3(23): 22–24.

Lowbury EJL, Ayliffe GAJ, Geddes AM and Williams JD (1992) *Control of Hospital Infection – A Practical Handbook*, 3rd Edition. London: Chapman & Hall.

MacKenzie I (1988) Preoperative skin preparation. Surgical outcome. Symposium on antiseptics and surgical patients. *Journal of Hospital Infection* 11 April, (Supplement B), 27–32.

Seropian R and Reynolds B (1971) Wound infection after pre-operative depilatory versus razor preparation. *American Journal of Surgery* 121, March, 251–253.

Shanson DC (1983) *Microbiology in Clinical Practice*, 2nd Edition. London: Wright.

9 POSTOPERATIVE CARE

Definition The period which follows surgical intervention.

Aims (a) Recognise and prevent factors which could contribute to a patient acquiring an infection.

(b) Patient should be nursed in the greatest comfort and encouraged to participate in his/her own care until complete recovery is affected.

Broad Principles

1. The environment should be clean, well ventilated and maintained (Ayliffe 1991).

2. All equipment should be well maintained, clean, disinfected or sterilised in accordance with local agreed policies (Ayliffe et al. 1992).

3. Linen should not be a source of cross-infection, therefore patients should be nursed in clean bedding (O'Brien 1986).

4. All invasive and wound dressing procedures should be carried out applying the principles of asepsis (*see* Principle No. 5).

5. Accumulating fluid in or around a wound should not contribute to patients developing an infection. A continuous, closed circuit wound drainage may therefore be necessary (Alderman 1989). Such drainage systems should be removed as soon as possible to reduce further the risk of infection (Ayliffe et al. 1992).

6. To avoid contamination, a drained wound should be dressed separately from the primary wound (Moir-Bussy 1986).

7. The patient should be pain-free, to reduce pressure on an unhealed wound (Egbert et al. 1964).

8. Used waste and equipment should be dealt with in accordance with local agreed policy (Collins and Josse 1990).

9. Staff should be able to identify any signs and symptoms, which could indicate a wound infection, and take appropriate action.

References

Ayliffe GAJ, Collins BJ and Taylor LJ (1991) *Hospital Acquired Infection. Principles and Prevention*, 2nd Edition. Guildford: Butterworth Heinemann Ltd.

Ayliffe GAJ, Lowbury EJL, Geddes ALM and Williams JD (1992) *Control of Hospital Infection – A Practical Handbook*, 3rd Edition. London: Chapman & Hall.

Alderman C (1989) Wound drainage. *Nursing Standard* 35(3): 34–6.

Collins BJ and Josse ED (1990) The Patient's Environment. In: Worsley MA, Ward KA and Parker L (eds) *Infection Control Guidelines for Nursing Care*. Livingston: ICNA/Surgikos.

Egbert LD, Battet GE, Welch CE and Bartlett MK (1964) Reduction of post-operative pain by encouragement and instruction of patient. *New England Journal of Medicine* 270(16): 285–87.

Moir-Bussy B (1986) The surgical wound. *Nursing* 3(3): 92–94.

O'Brien K (1986) Post-operative wound infection. *Nursing* 3(5): 178–186.

10 ORAL CARE

Definition The term is used to describe the care of the patient in relation to oral cleanliness.

Aims (a) To achieve and maintain oral cleanliness.
(b) To prevent infection, plaque and oral disease.

Broad Principles

1. To prevent cross-infection, protective clothing, such as gloves, should be worn when in contact with oral secretions (Ayliffe et al. 1992).

2. Dental plaque should be removed preferably with a tooth brush (Meckstroth 1989).

3. Dentures should be removed and cleaned regularly to prevent build up of debris.

4. The mouth should be assessed for signs of infection, dryness and odour (Hayes 1989).

5. To prevent cross-infection, equipment, if used, should be single-use or decontaminated between patients.

6. Equipment used should also be designed for maximum efficiency, e.g. toothbrushes should be small-headed and used in conjunction with a fluoride toothpaste (Gibbons 1983).

References

Ayliffe GAJ, Lowbury EJL, Geddes AM and Williams JD (1992) *Control of Hospital Infection – A Practical Handbook*, 3rd Edition. London: Chapman & Hall.

Gibbons DE (1983) Mouth care procedures. *Nursing Times* 79(7): 30.

Hayes B (1989) Oral hygiene – Theory v. practice. *Nursing Review* 7(3/4): 23–24.

Meckstroth RL (1989) Improving quality and efficiency in oral hygiene. *Journal of Gerontological Nursing* 15(6): 38–42.

11 TRACHEAL CARE

Definition A term used to describe any procedure used in the management of patients with either tracheostomy or endotracheal tubes.

Aims
1. To maintain a patient's airway.
2. To prevent infection.
3. To provide optimal healing conditions for patients with tracheostomies.

Broad Principles

1. Principles of handwashing (*see* Principle No. 2) and asepsis (*see* Principle No. 5) should apply for all tracheal care.

2. Trauma should be minimised during the insertion and handling of the tracheostomy and endotracheal tube (Stevenson 1990).

3. Protective clothing, i.e. plastic disposable gloves and apron, should be worn while tracheal care is being undertaken to reduce the risk of cross-infection to both the patient and carer. Consideration should be given to the wearing of masks if the patient has a known communicable disease such as open pulmonary tuberculosis (Stevenson 1990).

4. Tracheostomy and endotracheal tubes should be kept free of secretions by regular cleaning and suction (Caine and Bufalino 1988).

5. The skin around the stoma should be kept clean and dry and secretions removed as necessary to prevent excoriation (Pritchard and Mallet 1992).

6. Tracheostomy stoma site should be assessed for signs of healing or the presence of infection (Caine and Bufalino 1988).

7. Sterile suction catheters should be used for the aspiration of bronchial secretions to reduce the risk of infection (Ayliffe et al. 1992).

8. Contaminated clinical waste should be removed from the clinical area as soon as practicable (Collins and Josse 1990).

9. A decontamination and maintenance programme is required for the suction equipment both while it is in use and between each patient (Collins 1986, Creamer 1993).

References

Ayliffe GAJ, Lowbury EJL, Geddes AM and Williams JD (1992) *Control of Hospital Infection – A Practical Handbook*, 3rd Edition. London: Chapman & Hall.

Caine RM and Bufalino PM (1988) *Critically Ill. Adults: Nursing Care Planning Guides.* Baltimore: Williams & Wilkins.

Collins BJ (1986) Respiratory assistance – Care of equipment. *Intensive Care Nursing* 1(3): 138–143.

Collins BJ and Josse ED (1990) The Patient's Environment. In: Worsley MA, Ward KA and Parker L (eds) *Infection Control Guidelines for Nursing Care.* Livingston: ICNA/Surgikos.

Creamer E (1993) Decontamination quality. *Nursing Times* 89(36) The Journal of Infection Control Nursing, 65–68.

Stevenson G (1990) Nosocomial Respiratory Infection. In: Worsley MA, Ward KA and Parker L (eds) *Infection Control Guidelines for Nursing Care.* Livingston: ICNA/Surgikos.

Prichard, AP and Mallett J (1992) *Royal Marsden Hospital Manual of Clinical Nursing Procedures*, 3rd Edition. Oxford: Blackwell Scientific Publications.

12 CLINICAL WASTE

Definition The term is used to describe any clinical waste which unless rendered safe may prove to be hazardous to any person coming into contact with it, for example

- Waste which consists wholly or partly of human or animal tissue/blood/other body fluids.
- Swabs or dressings.
- Syringes, needles or other sharp instruments.
- Microbiological cultures and potentially infected waste from the Pathology Department.
- Certain pharmaceutical products and chemical waste (Health & Safety Commission 1992).

Aim To safeguard the general public and staff from hazardous clinical waste.

Broad Principles

1. All staff who work in areas where clinical waste arises should receive instructions in waste handling, segregation, storage and disposal procedures (Health & Safety Commission 1992).

2. There should be a standardised approach to the segregation, storage and disposal of waste at the point of generation, i.e. yellow plastic bags for waste that must be incinerated (Health & Safety Commission 1992).

3. Clinical waste bags should be robust enough to fulfil their function, i.e. designed and manufactured in accordance with the standards

set out by the NHS Supplies Authority or an equivalent standard (Health & Safety Commission 1992).

4. Spillage from bags should be avoided, therefore they should be replaced daily or when three quarters full.

5. Bags should always be securely tied at the neck using a method which does not injure the handler (London Waste Regulation Authority 1989).

6. Bags should be labelled with the source of the waste (Health & Safety Commission 1992).

7. Clinical waste should be transported safely in a cleaned or disinfected vehicle designated for that task (London Waste Regulation Authority 1989).

8. Waste should be stored safely in such a manner as to prevent
   (a) corrosion or wear of container;
   (b) accidental spillage or leakage.
   (c) accident or weather destroying the bags.
   (d) waste blowing away or falling while being stored.
   (e) Scavenging by vandals, animals, pests.
   (Department of the Environment 1991)

9. Used sharps must be stored in such a manner as to prevent injury or cross-infection to the hospital staff and general public (i.e. British Standard Specification for Sharps Containers BS 7320).

10. It should be the personal responsibility of individuals using sharps to ensure that they have adequate resources to dispose of the clinical waste safely (British Medical Association 1990).

11. All personnel involved in the disposal of clinical waste should wear protective clothing as identified in employer's clinical waste policy and by Control of Substances Hazardous to Health (COSHH) assessment (Health and Safety Commission 1992).

12. Any health care staff who sustains an injury while dealing with clinical waste must seek immediate help in accordance with local agreed policies.

References

Department of the Environment (1991) *Waste Management – The Duty of Care. A Code of Practice, issued in accordance with Environmental Protection Act 1990.* London: HMSO.

Health and Safety Commission (1992) *Health Services Advisory Committee. The Safe Disposal of Clinical Waste.* London: HMSO.

London Waste Regulation Authority (1989) *Guidelines for the Segregation, Handling and Transport of Clinical Waste.* London: London Waste Regulation Authority.

British Medical Association (1990) *A Code of Practice for the Safe Use and Disposal of Sharps.* London: BMA.

The Control of Substances Hazardous to Health (COSHH) Regulations, 1992. London: HMSO.

13 LINEN

Definition A service which is developed to process used linen.

Aim To prevent linen from becoming a cross-infection hazard.

Broad Principles

(a) COLLECTION OF LINEN

1. Aerosol dispersal of organisms should be prevented by handling used linen with minimum agitation (Bennet and Brachman 1992).

2. Local policies should reflect national guidelines (DHSS 1987).

3. The used linen should be categorised and placed in appropriate colour coded bags in accordance with the locally agreed policy (Ayliffe et al. 1992).

4. Effective handwashing should always follow the handling of used linen (Sanderson and Weisser 1992).

5. Staff involved in the handling of linen at the point of use should undergo training to raise awareness of the importance of correct bagging procedures and of the prevention of extraneous items from being collected with the linen (Ayliffe et al. 1992).

(b) STORAGE

1. Linen classed as infected should remain in secure storage until collection (DHSS 1987).

(c) TRANSPORTATION

1. During transportation used linen should remain securely contained in the appropriate colour coded bags (DHSS 1987).